Mindful Living Unleashed: Your Ultimate Guide to a Tranquil Day Amidst Chaos.

Lois D. Kroger

INTRODUCTION.

Finding a quiet time in the busyness of our modern life often seems like a distant dream. The incessant stream of information, obligations, and the unrelenting speed of everyday activities can cause us to feel overburdened and disengaged from our health. The idea of mindfulness seems as a ray of hope in this turbulent environment, providing a method to find peace in the middle of the storm.

"Mindful Living Unleashed" is an invitation to set out on a path of self-discovery and purposeful living, not just a manual. The secret of mindfulness's efficacy is its capacity to ground us in the now and now, enabling us to fully experience and value every aspect of our lives. We will explore the enigmas surrounding mindfulness in the upcoming chapters and acquire useful tools to bring peace of mind into our daily lives.

The goal of this book is to interact with reality more intentionally and consciously rather than to run away from it. The introduction lays the groundwork and invites you to consider all of the opportunities that mindful living presents. It is an opportunity to delve into the depths of your awareness, take a step back from the chaos, and re-establish a connection with your true self.

Through the next few chapters, we'll learn about mindful morning routines that help provide a peaceful start to the day, workplace mindfulness practices, and even techniques to appreciate the act of eating itself. All of the sections—from deliberate periods of retreat to mindful movement—offer useful insights that you can easily incorporate into your everyday routine.

The trip becomes a way of life that never ends—it doesn't stop with the last chapter. "Mindful Living Unleashed" is a journey through the present moment that leads to regaining inner peace and appreciating life to the fullest. It is not a destination. So let's go off on this life-changing journey together, one peaceful moment at a time, unleashing the power of mindful living.

CHAPTER 1.
The Power of Mindfulness.

The power of mindfulness manifests as a transformational force amid the ever-accelerating pace of modern life, providing comfort and resilience in the face of chaos. Fundamentally, mindfulness is the practice of being present, of engaging with the here and now with awareness and without the burden of regrets from the past or fears about the future.

The capacity of mindfulness to increase consciousness is its main strength. It's a deft maneuver through the maze of feelings, ideas, and outside influences that enables us to look at things objectively. We gain a deep grasp of the environment around us, our responses, and ourselves via this monitoring.

We develop an awareness of the present moment through purposeful activities like body scans, mindful breathing, and meditation. This elevated consciousness turns into a haven, a haven from the turbulent currents of worry and diversion. We find a tranquility reservoir in the simplicity of thoughtful moments, which we may tap into during life's storms.

<u>The advantages of mindfulness in our life are numerous and include:</u>

1. Reduction of Stress: Mindfulness is a potent remedy for stress, offering a haven where the mind may escape the pressures of everyday existence.

2. Enhanced Mental Clarity: Mindfulness improves cognitive function by helping us focus on the here and now, which facilitates better decision-making and problem-solving.

3. Emotional Regulation: We can learn to observe our feelings without becoming overwhelmed by them by cultivating mindful awareness, which promotes emotional resilience.

4. Improved Well-Being: Consistent mindfulness exercises have been connected to enhanced general well-being, which includes more restful sleep, self-awareness, and happier emotions.

5. Greater Compassion: Mindfulness cultivates a compassionate perspective toward ourselves as well as others, enabling us to have a kinder and more understanding relationship with our ideas and deeds.

Through the practice of mindfulness, we can bring about a significant transformation in the way we see and manage the complexities of our lives, bringing about a calmness that surpasses the disorderliness of the outside world.

CHAPTER 2.
Morning Rituals for a Calm Start.

Establishing peaceful morning routines sets the tone for the day. Start with a gradual waking rather than a startling burst of alarms. Alternatively, let ambient lighting or relaxing music lead you into awareness. Take some time to practice mindfulness before the outside world gets in. Make time in the early morning hours for peace, whether it be by gratitude meditation, deep breathing, or thoughtful thoughts. Consider eating a healthy breakfast as a kind of self-care for your body.

Include exercise in your morning routine, whether it be yoga, stretching, or a quick stroll. This prepares the mind for the upcoming day and revitalizes the body. Accept the influence of establishing intentions. Make sure that your daily objectives are clear and that you have a purpose. Think of journaling as a contemplative exercise where you write down your goals and ideas.

In the early hours, try to avoid using digital gadgets too much. Instead, spend time creating art, reading a book, or spending time with loved ones. Developing a daily ritual that works as an anchor for your day, offers steadiness in an uncertain world. These rituals serve as flexible foundations rather than strict guidelines, adjusting to your needs and promoting equilibrium and serenity.

CHAPTER 3.
Mindful Work: Navigating Stress with Ease.

The secret to working mindfully is knowing when to give in to stress. Start by setting up an atmosphere in your office that is attentive and promotes calmness and concentration. Divide the day into digestible chunks and include brief, conscious breaks to help you refocus. Engage in deep breathing techniques to help you center yourself in stressful situations and maintain a cool, collected demeanor.

The idea of mindful work emerges as a guiding light in the hectic world of work, where expectations and deadlines loom constantly. This practice helps people manage stress and maintain a sense of balance in their professional lives.

- **Establishing a Mindful Workspace:** Start by designing a setting that encourages calmness and concentration. To promote peace, get rid of extraneous clutter, add natural features, and personalize the area. The basis for a thoughtful approach to work is this physical setting.

- **Mindfully Dividing the Day:** Divide your workday into digestible chunks. Accept the benefits of taking mindful breaks, getting up from your desk to stretch, taking a little breather, or practicing mindfulness. These breaks act as reset buttons, keeping tension from building up and refocusing your attention.

- **Breathing for Calm:** Pay attention to your breath whenever stress creeps in. Engage in deep breathing techniques to help you stay grounded in the here and now. By concentrating on your breathing, you can both relax and build a defense against the hectic demands of the office.

- **Single-tasking vs. Multitasking:** Accept single-tasking and dispel the illusion of multitasking. Focus entirely on one job at a time to encourage a more in-depth and meaningful interaction. This thoughtful approach lessens the mental strain that comes with juggling several obligations while increasing efficiency.

- **Setting and Creating Realistic Objectives:** Setting and achieving realistic objectives is a component of mindful work. Break down more difficult tasks into smaller, more manageable segments. Establish defined priorities to ensure that your efforts are aligned with the overarching objectives. This strategic move boosts productivity while lowering stress.

- **Mindful Engagement in Work Activities:** Apply mindfulness to all aspects of your work life, including email correspondence, meeting participation, and project management. Develop a heightened awareness of the current moment, give your whole attention to the activity at hand, and be present. This deliberate participation helps you feel fulfilled and purposeful in your work.

- **Developing a Mindful Attitude:** Take a thoughtful approach to problems. Consider them as learning opportunities rather than sources of tension. By changing your viewpoint, you can turn challenges into learning opportunities and develop adaptability and resilience in the face of job expectations.

- **Gratitude Moments:** Spread gratitude-filled moments throughout your workweek. Reward both minor and major achievements with thanks for the work accomplished. This exercise combats the propensity to become fixated on stressors and instills a positive outlook.

- **Setting good Boundaries:** By establishing boundaries, you can keep a good work-life balance. Make a clear distinction between your job and personal time to prevent work from creeping into your free time. Setting these limits helps people stay healthy generally and avoids burnout.

The aim of adopting mindful work is to change your relationship with stress rather than completely remove it. You can handle the rigors of your work life with grace, resiliency, and ease if you engage in these mindful practices.

CHAPTER 4.

Mindful Eating: Savoring Every Bite.

The practice of mindful eating emerges as a revolutionary approach to sustenance, urging people to savor every bite with intention and awareness in a society where meals are frequently rushed and taken on the move. The food on your plate is only one aspect of mindful eating; it's a comprehensive experience that includes all of the senses and strengthens the bond between your body and mind.

- **Savoring the Present:** The first step towards mindful eating is making a conscious effort to focus entirely on the here and now. Spend some time appreciating the flavors, textures, and colors of your food when you sit down to eat. Give your senses their complete attention and lose yourself in the process of giving your body nourishment.

- **Slowing Down the Pace:** Mindful eating promotes a slower, more deliberate pace in a society where people are used to living fast-paced lives. Set electronics aside, disable any outside distractions, and concentrate on eating. By eating more slowly, you allow your body to communicate when it is full, which helps with digestion and keeps you from overeating.

- **Chewing with Awareness:** Mindful eating places a strong emphasis on the significance of mindfully chewing each bite. As you chew, take note of the flavors and textures and let the digestion process start in your mouth. This easy gesture not only makes your meal more enjoyable but also promotes healthy digestion.

<u>Advantages of Intentional Eating:</u>

1. Better Digestion: You can improve your digestion and minimize your risk of indigestion and bloating by chewing your food well and eating more slowly.

2. Enhanced Taste Sensitivity: Eating mindfully makes you more sensitive to flavor, which enables you to completely enjoy and savor the variety of flavors in your food.

3. Weight Management: Eating more slowly gives the body more time to sense fullness, which lowers the chance of overindulging and helps with weight management objectives.

4. Greater Satisfaction: Meals provide greater physical and emotional fulfillment when you take time to savor each bite. A better connection with food is facilitated by this sense of fulfillment.

5. Heightened Awareness of Hunger and Fullness: Eating mindfully helps you become more aware of your body's signals of hunger and fullness, so you can recognize when you're truly hungry and stop yourself from overindulging in snacks.

6. Less Emotional Eating: attentive eating encourages a more attentive reaction to stress and

emotions by raising awareness of the eating
process. This breaks the cycle of emotional eating.

7. Connection to Food Sources: By encouraging a
closer relationship with the places your food comes
from, mindful eating helps you feel grateful for the
natural sustenance that nature provides.

8. Development of Mindful Habits: As you become
more aware of your body's demands, mindful eating
practices influence other areas of your life in addition
to meals.

In a culture where people are driven by their
schedules, making mindful eating a part of your
everyday routine provides a break—an opportunity
to rediscover the joys of food and cultivate a positive
relationship with it. One meal at a time, you set out
on a path to greater well-being as you mindfully
relish each bite.

CHAPTER 5.
Finding Tranquility in Movement: Mindful Exercise.

In the search for well-being, the concept of mindful exercise develops as a transformative approach to physical activity—one that transcends the basic act of movement and enables individuals to find calm in the rhythm of their bodies. Mindful exercise is a mindful and intentional involvement with physical activity, building a deep connection between the mind and the body. As you embark on this journey, each movement becomes a meditative experience, a study of the present moment via the language of the body.

Mindful Movement Practices:

1. Yoga: Embrace the ancient practice of yoga, where breath and movement connect to create a harmonic flow. From mild stretches to powerful positions, yoga develops a mindful connection with the body and breath.

2. Tai Chi: This martial art is characterized by calm, flowing movements that develop balance, flexibility, and mental focus. Tai Chi is a movement meditation, that enables practitioners to be present in each elegant action.

3. Walking Meditation: Transform your daily stroll into a mindful activity by paying attention to each step, the sensation of your feet contacting the earth, and the rhythm of your breath. Walking becomes a meditative discipline, grounding you in the present moment.

4. Pilates: Focus on regulated exercises that activate the core, developing strength, flexibility, and body awareness. Pilates offers a thoughtful approach to each exercise, establishing a deeper connection with the body's movements.

5. Dance: Whether in a scheduled class or a spontaneous solo dance practice, mindful dancing entails being fully present in the movement, allowing the music to direct your body with intention and expression.

<u>Benefits of Mindful Exercise:</u>

1. Enhanced Mind-Body link: Mindful exercise strengthens the link between your physical and mental states. By being fully present in each movement, you create a heightened awareness of your body's potential and limitations.

2. Stress Reduction: Engaging in mindful exercise provides a respite from the responsibilities of daily life. The focused concentration on movement and breath promotes relaxation, lowering stress and tension.

3. Improved Concentration: The purposeful focus required in mindful exercise spills over into daily life, boosting your capacity to concentrate and stay present in varied tasks.

4. Increased Flexibility: Many mindful movement practices, such as yoga and Pilates, develop flexibility through controlled and focused stretching, contributing to a greater range of motion.

5. Balanced Emotions: Mindful exercise increases the release of endorphins, generating a happy mood and a sense of emotional balance.

6. Mindful Breathing: Incorporating breath awareness during exercise promotes respiratory function and mindfulness. Breath becomes a guide, aligning with movements for a more coordinated and aware experience.

7. Improved Posture: Mindful movement activities frequently emphasize optimal alignment and body awareness, contributing to improved posture and reduced strain on muscles and joints.

8. Enhanced Body Image: By creating a good and conscious relationship with your body through exercise, you build a better body image and appreciation for what your body can achieve.

9. Better Sleep: Regular engagement in mindful exercise has been associated with enhanced sleep quality, leading to overall well-being.

10. Joyful Connection to Movement: Mindful exercise turns physical activity from a routine task to a source of joy and self-expression. Movement becomes a celebration of the body's possibilities and a source of self-care.

As you engage in mindful exercise, the advantages transcend beyond the physical sphere, penetrating your mental and emotional well-being. Each intentional movement becomes a step towards holistic health—a journey where calm is found in the attentive dance between body and mind.

CHAPTER 6.

Digital Detox: Unplugging for Inner Peace.

In a society dominated by screens and constant communication, the notion of a digital detox has become a strong cure to the stress and information overload that permeate our daily lives. Unplugging from digital devices is not just a short retreat; it's an intentional choice to restore inner serenity and nurture a deeper connection with the present moment. As you embark on a digital detox, you make space for mental clarity, true connection, and a profound sense of well-being.

Understanding the Need for a Digital Detox:

The persistent buzzing of notifications, the steady flood of emails, and the draw of social media may overwhelm our senses, leaving us in a perpetual state of distraction. A digital detox is a deliberate break from this digital cacophony, allowing for a reset and a return to a more thoughtful way of living.

Benefits of a Digital Detox:

1. Improved Mental Well-being: Disconnecting from digital gadgets minimizes the mental clutter associated with frequent information consumption. This respite helps your mind to relax, providing mental clarity and a sensation of tranquility.

2. Enhanced Focus and Productivity: A digital detox provides relief from the continuous disruptions that impede focus. With fewer distractions, you may put your energy into projects with more concentration and efficiency.

3. Deeper Connection to the Present Moment: Without the constant tug of notifications, you may fully immerse yourself in the present moment. This heightened awareness produces a deeper experience of life outside the digital domain.

4. Stress Reduction: The continual flood of information and the pressure to stay connected lead to stress. A digital detox gives relief, allowing stress levels to reduce as you withdraw and prioritize self-care.

5. Quality Sleep: The blue light emitted by devices can interrupt sleep patterns. By unplugging before bedtime, you promote greater sleep quality, adding to overall well-being.

6. Authentic Human Connection: Digital communication, while convenient, frequently lacks the depth of face-to-face encounters. A digital detox enables meaningful, in-person contacts, building a sense of community and support.

7. Enhanced Creativity: Constant digital stimulus might inhibit creativity. During a digital detox, your mind is free to wander, leading to improved inspiration and new thinking.

8. Reduced Anxiety: The fear of missing out (FOMO) and the frequent comparison on social media platforms add to anxiety. A digital detox alleviates these stresses, allowing for a more positive outlook.

<u>Digital Detox Exercise</u>:

1. Unplug for a Day: Designate a day to entirely unplug from all digital gadgets. Use this time to indulge in activities that bring you joy and relaxation, whether it's reading a book, spending time in nature, or performing a hobby.

2. Tech-Free Mealtime: Create a sacred place during meals by refraining from using digital devices. Instead, consume each bite carefully, engage in conversation, or enjoy the quietude of your surroundings.

3. Social Media Sabbatical: Take a sabbatical from social media for a specified duration. Use this time to reassess your relationship with these platforms and to focus on more meaningful contacts in the offline world.

4. Mindful Screen Time: When necessary, be thoughtful about your screen time. Set specific periods for reading emails or social media, and use applications or features that measure and limit your daily usage.

5. Nature Walk Without Devices: Embark on a nature walk without any digital devices. Allow yourself to be fully present in nature, taking in the sights, sounds, and sensations without the filter of a screen.

A digital detox is not about rejecting technology totally but rather about establishing a healthy and thoughtful connection with it. By implementing these digital detox exercises into your routine, you make space for inner calm, true connection, and a more intentional way of living.

CHAPTER 7.
Mindful Moments: Creating Micro-Retreats in Your Day.

In the fast-paced cadence of modern life, where obligations and distractions abound, the concept of establishing micro-retreats through thoughtful moments becomes a powerful technique for building serenity and balance. These micro-retreats are not grandiose expeditions to exotic places but intentional pauses woven into the fabric of your day, allowing you to recharge, refocus, and reconnect with a sense of peace in the daily scurry.

Creating Micro-Retreats:

1. Breath Awareness Breaks: Take a few minutes at various points throughout your day to engage in concentrated breath awareness. Inhale deeply, hold for a time and exhale gently. This simple technique anchors you in the present, allowing a little respite from the continual stream of ideas.

2. Mindful Walking: Transform everyday walks into mindful journeys. Pay attention to each stride, the sensation of your feet touching the earth, and the rhythm of your breath. Whether it's a stroll around the office or a little outside walk, this exercise brings a sense of retreat into the commonplace.

3. Five Senses Check-In: Ground yourself in the present moment by engaging your senses. Take time to observe five things you can see, four things you can touch, three things you can hear, two things you can smell, and one item you can taste. This sensory check-in gives a rapid and effective retreat into mindfulness.

4. Nature Connection: Stepping outside, even for a few minutes, can be a mini-retreat in itself. Immerse yourself in nature, feel the sun on your skin, listen to the sounds of birds or leaves rustling, and take in the colors surrounding you. Nature's simplicity delivers a profound reset.

5. Gratitude Pause: Pause and think about three things you're grateful for at that exact moment. Whether it's a supportive coworker, a moment of serenity, or a tiny success, this thankfulness exercise redirects your emphasis toward the positive.

Benefits of Micro-Retreats:

1. Stress Reduction: Micro-retreats work as stress-relieving interludes, breaking the cycle of stress and offering moments of calm throughout the day. This proactive strategy helps prevent stress from mounting.

2. Improved Focus: Taking intentional breaks boosts your capacity to concentrate. After a micro-retreat, you return to work with renewed focus and clarity, potentially enhancing total productivity.

3. Emotional Regulation: Pausing for attentive moments allows you to examine and regulate your emotions. This awareness avoids reactive responses to stressors and increases emotional resilience.

4. Enhanced Well-being: Incorporating micro-retreats into your day leads to an overall sense of well-being. These moments of reprieve build mental and emotional equilibrium, boosting your quality of life.

5. Increased work: Contrary to the belief that breaks impede work, micro-retreats boost efficiency. They avoid fatigue, maintain a sustainable pace, and contribute to a more productive work atmosphere.

6. Mindful Decision-Making: Creating room for mindful moments enables you to approach decisions with greater awareness and discernment. This attentiveness leads to more thoughtful and well-informed choices.

7. Elevated Mood: Micro-retreats function as mood-boosting interludes. By taking minutes to center yourself, you create a good mindset and build resilience in the face of adversity.

In accepting these micro-retreats, you build a tapestry of self-care throughout your day. These intentional pauses act as an anchor, keeping you in the present moment and providing moments of consolation in the middle of life's demands. As you combine these practices, you create a mindful approach to living—one that understands the importance of tiny, intentional getaways in sustaining your well-being.

CHAPTER 8.
Evening Reflections: Gratitude and Relaxation.

As the day draws to a close, the practice of evening meditations provides a quiet entryway to gratitude and rest. It's an intentional pause, inviting you to unwind, acknowledge the day's experiences, and create a sense of appreciation. In the quiet minutes before sleep, engaging in evening meditations sets the stage for comfortable sleeping and creates a happy mood that stretches throughout the next day.

Evening Reflections Routine:

1. Gratitude Journaling: Dedicate a few moments to jot down three things you're grateful for during the day. Whether it's a simple act of kindness, a moment of joy, or an accomplishment, thankfulness writing redirects your emphasis toward positivity.

2. Mindful Breathing: Incorporate a brief mindful breathing exercise. Close your eyes, inhale deeply, hold for a time, then release gently. This focused breathwork soothes the nervous system and signals to your body that it's time to unwind.

3. Reviewing Achievements: Reflect on your accomplishments, no matter how modest. Acknowledge the chores you did, problems you overcame, or moments of personal progress. This positive reflection instills a sense of fulfillment.

4. Digital Detox: Create a boundary between your evening reflections and digital devices. Avoid screen time at least 30 minutes before bedtime to reduce exposure to blue light, supporting better sleep quality.

5. Relaxing Activities: Engage in a peaceful activity such as reading a book, listening to soothing music, or practicing gentle stretches. These activities signal to your body that it's time to transition into a state of relaxation.

Importance of Evening Reflections:

1. Improved Sleep Quality: Engaging in evening meditations and relaxation activities indicates to your body that it's time to wind down, contributing to enhanced sleep quality and overall restfulness.

2. Positive mentality: Gratitude blogging and reflecting on achievements build a positive mentality, creating a sense of happiness and pleasure.

3. Stress Reduction: Evening meditations serve as a release valve for the day's stressors. By accepting challenges and expressing thankfulness, you create mental space for relaxing.

4. Enhanced Self-Awareness: Regular introspection develops self-awareness. It allows you to detect trends in your thoughts and behaviors, enabling personal growth and a greater awareness of yourself.

5. Cultivation of Gratitude: Gratitude writing promotes a habit of appreciation. By continually noticing the wonderful aspects of your day, you build a mentality of thankfulness that transcends beyond the evening thoughts.

6. conscious shift: Evening meditations give a conscious shift from the busyness of the day to a state of calm. This intentional adjustment prepares your mind for a restful night's sleep.

As you accept the practice of evening meditations, it becomes a quiet ritual—a pleasant way to bid farewell to the day and welcome the serenity of the night. Through gratitude and relaxation, you create a healthy bridge between the activities of the day and the peacefulness of the evening, encouraging a sense of balance and well-being.

CHAPTER 9.
Mindful Sleep Practices: Drifting into Serenity.

As the night approaches, embracing mindful sleep practices becomes a sacred journey into serenity—a deliberate transition from wakefulness to rest. These practices are not mere routines but intentional rituals that invite you to release the day's tensions, quiet the mind, and embrace the gentle embrace of sleep. By weaving mindfulness into your bedtime routine, you set the stage for a peaceful and rejuvenating night's rest.

Mindful Sleep Practices:

1. Screen Time Reduction: Minimize exposure to screens at least 30 minutes before bedtime. The blue light emitted from devices can disrupt melatonin production, hindering the body's natural sleep-wake cycle.

2. Mindful Breathing: Engage in mindful breathing exercises as you settle into bed. Inhale deeply, allowing your breath to fill your lungs, hold for a moment, and exhale slowly. This intentional breathwork signals to your body that it's time to relax.

3. Body Scan Meditation: Conduct a gentle body scan meditation, starting from your toes and gradually moving up to the crown of your head. Bring awareness to each part of your body, releasing tension and promoting a sense of ease.

4. Gratitude Reflection: Take a moment to reflect on three things you're grateful for from the day. Focusing on positive aspects cultivates a sense of contentment, contributing to a more relaxed mindset.

5. Create a Relaxing Environment: Ensure your sleep space is conducive to relaxation. Dim the lights, keep the room cool, and create a soothing atmosphere with calming scents or gentle background noise.

6. Restrict Stimulants: steer clear of stimulants right before bedtime, including caffeine and large meals. If needed, choose a light snack that will help you fall asleep.

7. Guided Imagery: Visualize a serene and peaceful place as you lie in bed. Whether it's a calming beach, a tranquil forest, or a cozy room, guided imagery helps shift your focus away from daily stressors.

Benefits of Mindful Sleep Practices:

1. Improved Sleep Quality: Mindful sleep practices contribute to improved sleep quality by signaling to your body that it's time to unwind and transition into restful sleep.

2. Stress Reduction: Engaging in calming practices before bedtime helps release accumulated stress, promoting a sense of calm that carries into your sleep.

3. Enhanced Relaxation: Mindful breathing, body scans, and guided imagery foster a state of relaxation, allowing you to let go of the day's tensions and embrace a serene mindset.

4. Natural Sleep Induction: By creating a bedtime routine that prioritizes mindfulness, you enhance your body's natural sleep induction processes, making it easier to drift into restful sleep.

5. Mind-Body Connection: These practices deepen the connection between your mind and body, aligning them in a harmonious state that supports restorative sleep.

6. Consistent Sleep Patterns: Establishing mindful sleep practices helps regulate your sleep patterns, contributing to a more consistent and predictable nightly routine.

7. Morning Wakefulness: A restful night sets the foundation for a refreshed morning. Mindful sleep practices contribute to waking up with a clear mind and increased energy.

In weaving these mindful sleep practices into your nightly routine, bedtime becomes more than a necessity—it transforms into a sanctuary for serenity and rejuvenation. By embracing mindfulness in the moments leading up to sleep, you embark on a journey into the restorative realms of the night, awakening with a renewed sense of well-being each morning.

CHAPTER 10.
Integrating Mindfulness into Daily Life.

Integrating mindfulness into daily life is a transforming journey that entails weaving awareness into the fabric of your routine. It's not about carving out isolated moments for mindfulness but injecting presence into every activity, conversation, and experience. By cultivating this deliberate awareness, you welcome a sense of serenity, clarity, and purpose into each passing moment.

Practical Ways to Integrate Mindfulness.

1. Morning Mindfulness Routine: Begin your day with a few moments of mindfulness. Whether through mindful breathing, a short meditation, or a gratitude reflection, establish a positive tone for the day ahead.

2. Mindful Eating: Slow down and savor each bite throughout meals. Pay attention to the flavors, textures, and experiences. This thoughtful approach not only enriches the meal experience but also supports good digestion.

3. Breath Awareness Breaks: Take small breaks throughout the day to participate in concentrated breath awareness. Inhale deeply, hold for a time and exhale gently. These tiny mindful breaks anchor you in the present moment.

4. Single-Tasking: Embrace single-tasking over multitasking. Focus your concentration totally on one task at a time, whether it's work-related, a domestic chore, or a personal project. This method promotes efficiency and mindfulness.

5. thoughtful Walking: Transform your walks into thoughtful journeys. Pay attention to each stride, the sensation of your feet touching the earth, and the rhythm of your breath. Walking becomes a meditative practice.

6. Technology Awareness: Consciously engage with technology. Set boundaries for screen time, minimize mindless scrolling, and be present during virtual interactions. Mindful technology use develops a healthier connection with devices.

7. Mindful Listening: Practice active and empathic listening throughout interactions. Fully engage with the speaker, set aside judgments, and answer with thoughtful thinking. Mindful listening improves bonds.

8. Mindful Transitions: Infuse attention into transitional periods. Whether it's transitioning between work, locations, or hobbies, take a breath and bring your consciousness to the present before moving forward.

<u>Rewards of Integrating Mindfulness:</u>

1. Stress Reduction: Mindfulness helps interrupt the cycle of stress by developing a calm and centered mentality, allowing you to negotiate problems with more ease.

2. Improved Focus and Concentration: By teaching your mind to be present, mindfulness promotes focus and concentration, leading to enhanced productivity and efficiency.

3. Emotional Regulation: Mindfulness cultivates emotional resilience. It provides a room to watch and respond to emotions with greater awareness, preventing reactive responses.

4. Enhanced Well-being: Integrating mindfulness into daily living adds to overall well-being. It encourages a good outlook, decreases worry, and fosters a sense of contentment.

5. Better Decision-Making: Mindfulness sharpens cognitive capacities and enhances clarity of thought. This, in turn, fosters more thoughtful and well-informed decision-making.

6. Deeper bonds: Mindful presence in conversations enhances bonds with others. It creates empathy, understanding, and a more meaningful relationship with those around you.

7. Increased Self-Awareness: Mindfulness increases self-reflection and self-awareness. By observing thoughts and behaviors without judgment, you get insights into your patterns and inclinations.

8. Heightened Appreciation: creating mindfulness allows you to appreciate the richness of each moment, finding joy in simple pleasures, and creating a gratitude-filled outlook.

As you integrate mindfulness into your regular life, it becomes a way of being rather than a discipline isolated to specific moments. This deliberate presence transforms mundane activities into chances for connection, growth, and a better understanding of the beautiful fabric of life.

CONCLUSION.

To sum up, the path of mindfulness involves a deep examination of the present moment and a deliberate decision to weave awareness into the fabric of everyday existence. Being aware is a way of being that penetrates every activity and encounter, from the peaceful breaths that greet the day to the contemplative moments that precede sleep.

By incorporating mindfulness into your daily practice, you take a revolutionary step that changes the way you interact with the outside world. Whether enjoying a meal's flavors, taking intentional walks, or just taking deep breaths during stressful times, mindfulness becomes a guiding partner that provides comfort, direction, and clarity.

This deliberate presence has numerous advantages, ranging from lowered stress and sharper focus to greater well-being and stronger bonds. A journey into the essence of every instant that passes is what mindfulness is, not some far-off place to get at. This trip is revealed with every step, breath, and heartbeat.

May this journey of mindfulness serve as a gentle reminder to appreciate the beauty in the small things, to face difficulties head-on, and to find peace in the ups and downs of life. May mindfulness be the note that balances your mind, body, and spirit in the symphony of life, producing a peaceful resonance that permeates everyday experiences.